PREGNANCY AND HEALTHY DIETS

FOODS TO AVOID DURING PREGNANCY: Comprehensive Guide to Navigating Safe and Healthy Eating for Expectant Mothers.

JOHN LYNN

Table of Contents:

INTRODUCTION

NOURISHING A HEALTHY PREGNANCY

Understanding the Impact of Diet on Pregnancy

Pregnancy is a transformational and delicate journey defined by significant physiological changes and milestones. Among the important aspects determining this trip, nutrition takes center stage. The introduction to "Foods to Avoid During Pregnancy" dives into the enormous influence that dietary choices have on the well-being of both the pregnant woman and her growing infant.

Embarking on a Nutritional Odyssey:
Nutrition and pregnancy refer to the nutrient intake and dietary planning during and after pregnancy. The mother's nutrition significantly impacts the child's health, including the risk of cancer, cardiovascular disease, hypertension, and diabetes. Inadequate or excessive nutrients can

cause malformations, medical problems, neurological disorders, and handicaps. Malnourished mothers are at a higher risk of birthweight issues, with an estimated 24% of babies born with lower weights. Personal habits like alcohol or caffeine consumption can also negatively impact the baby's development during early pregnancy. The introduction explores how a mother's nutrient and dietary decisions directly impact her unborn child's growth, development, and overall health.

Balancing Nutritional Needs:

Understanding the necessity of a balanced diet throughout pregnancy becomes crucial. This section digs into the many nutrients important for fetal growth, mother health, and the avoidance of problems. It unravels the secret of how a well-rounded diet may be a cornerstone for a good pregnancy, impacting everything from the baby's organ development to the mother's energy levels and emotions.

<u>**Importance of Safe Eating Practices**</u>
Safeguarding Maternal and Fetal Health:
The introduction highlights the vital significance that healthy eating choices have in preserving both mother and fetal health. It discusses the possible dangers associated with ingesting specific foods during pregnancy, ranging from foodborne diseases to exposure to hazardous chemicals. By identifying these dangers, pregnant moms are empowered to make educated decisions that emphasize the well-being of themselves and their unborn child.

Empowering informed decision-making:
Safe eating habits extend beyond merely avoiding particular foods. This part addresses the larger terrain of informed decision-making—considering food handling, storage, and preparation. It provides readers with the information they need to navigate shopping aisles, understand food labels, and make choices that align with the concepts of a balanced and safe pregnancy diet.

In essence, the introduction sets the stage for pregnant moms, caregivers, and those beginning the joyful adventure of pregnancy. It uncovers the significant influence of food on this transforming era, demonstrating the connection between nutrition, mother health, and fetal growth. As readers immerse themselves in the pages that follow, they are led on a nutritious journey, equipped with the information to make educated and health-conscious choices that celebrate the marvel of life.

Chapter 1

NAVIGATING THE FIRST TRIMESTER

The first trimester of pregnancy is an exciting yet potentially frightening time for expecting women. However, physical symptoms can be overwhelming. This article provides information on the body's changes, recommended foods for the first 13 weeks, and advice on managing illness.

Embarking on the First Trimester Journey:
Pregnancy dating starts four weeks into the first trimester, which includes the first 13 weeks of pregnancy. During this time, the body experiences a surge in pregnancy hormones, including estrogen and progesterone, which can cause nausea and morning sickness. Human chorionic gonadotropin (HCG) is also increasing, potentially causing nausea and frequent urination. Progesterone slows down muscle action, potentially leading to constipation. The first 13 weeks are crucial for

milk production, with the baby weighing around 1 ounce by the end of the trimester. The body is exhausted due to the significant work it is doing.

Managing morning sickness during pregnancy:

Morning sickness is common during the first trimester, but it can occur at any time of the day and can be triggered by various factors. Food aversions and nausea can also be linked to sickness. Strategies for managing nausea include avoiding empty stomachs, eating smaller meals more frequently, eating lower-fat meals, and drinking enough water. Eating foods that are easier for the body to digest, such as rice, applesauce, fresh fruit, and multigrain crackers, can help alleviate nausea. Some people may crave comfort foods, such as sweet potatoes or ice cream. A balanced diet is essential during pregnancy, with fruits and vegetables being consumed when feeling well and avoiding unhealthy foods when not feeling well. If nausea or food aversions persist, it is important to consult a prenatal practitioner. Cold foods, ginger, peppermint, lemon, and bland foods can help with nausea.

Exercise during first trimester:
Pregnancy-induced exercise is beneficial for both mother and baby, as long as it's safe and doesn't cause light-headedness, dizziness, or shakiness. The American College of Obstetricians and Gynecologists recommends 150 minutes of moderate-intensity activity per week, including cardio and strength training. Exercises include walking, swimming, strength training, stationary biking, yoga, and Pilates.

Critical Nutrients and Early Pregnancy
1. Folic Acid for Neural Tube Development:
Folic acid is a crucial nutrient for preparing the body for pregnancy, as it is the synthetic form of the vitamin folate. It is essential both pre- and post-conception, as deficiencies in folic acid can lead to neural tube defects (NTDs). Women who supplemented with 0.4 mg of folic acid three months before childbirth significantly reduced the risk of NTDs. Over 80 countries use the

fortification of certain foods with folic acid to decrease NTD rates. Folic acid is found in dietary supplements and fortified grains, such as breakfast cereal, bread, pasta, and rice. Folate is found mainly in dark green vegetables like broccoli, asparagus, and romaine lettuce, as well as other plant foods like avocado, beans, and oranges. The Centers for Disease Control and Prevention recommend that women of childbearing age who are capable of becoming pregnant consume 400 mcg of folic acid daily along with a diet that includes folate-rich foods.

2. **Iron for Blood Formation**:
Explanation: Iron promotes the increased blood volume required for both mother and baby.
Illustration: Opt for lean meats, legumes, and fortified cereals to satisfy iron needs.
Example: A beef stir-fry with colorful veggies supplies iron and important nutrients.

3. **Calcium for Bone Health**:
Approximately 30 grams (1.1 oz) of calcium are deposited throughout pregnancy, practically all

of it in the fetal skeleton. For women with poor calcium diets, there is low-quality data to indicate that calcium supplementation during pregnancy may lower the incidence of preeclampsia. Low-quality research also shows that calcium supplementation may lessen the likelihood of the woman delivering the baby before the 37th week of pregnancy (preterm delivery). The preventive impact of calcium supplementation is not obvious, and there is not enough excellent quality to study to advise ideal amounts and timing of calcium intake.

Explanation: Calcium is crucial for the baby's developing bones and teeth.
Illustration: Incorporate dairy products, fortified plant-based milk, and leafy greens.
Example: A smoothie with yogurt, kale, and almond milk is a calcium-rich choice.

4. **Protein for Tissue Development**:
Explanation: Proteins contribute to the development of the baby's tissues and organs.

Illustration: Include sources including eggs, chicken, fish, and legumes in your diet.

Example: Grilled fish with quinoa gives a protein-packed and healthy dinner.

5. **Vitamin and mineral supplements:**

Multiple micronutrient supplements taken with iron and folic acid may enhance pregnancy outcomes for mothers in low-income nations. These supplements minimize rates of low birth weight infants, small for gestational age newborns, and stillbirths in women who may not have many micronutrients in their typical diets. Undernourished women might benefit from having nutritional instruction sessions and balanced energy and protein supplements. A study indicated that nutritional education raised the mother's protein intake and helped the baby develop more within the womb. The balanced protein and energy supplement cut the risk of stillbirth and tiny newborns and boosted weight growth for both the mother and baby.

Foods to Limit for a Healthy Start

1. Caffeine Intake:

Caffeine consumption during pregnancy is linked to an increased risk of pregnancy loss and low birth weight. The European Food Safety Authority and the American Congress of Obstetricians and Gynecologists agree that habitual caffeine consumption up to 200 mg per day is safe for the fetus. The UK Food Standards Agency initially recommended limiting caffeine intake to less than 300 mg daily, but revised this to less than 200 mg in 2009. High caffeine intake during pregnancy may increase the risk of miscarriage and other negative pregnancy outcomes. A 2020 review questioned the safe levels proposed by the European Food Safety Authority, the American Congress of Obstetricians and Gynecologists, the National Health Service, and Dietary Guidelines for Americans, stating that current scientific evidence does not support moderate caffeine consumption during pregnancy as safe and advised pregnant women and women considering pregnancy to avoid caffeine entirely.

Explanation: High caffeine intake may be associated with an increased risk of miscarriage.
Illustration: Limit coffee, tea, and soda; opt for decaffeinated options.
Example: Herbal teas or decaf coffee can be satisfying alternatives.

2. **Alcohol**:

Fetal alcohol spectrum disorders, a group of conditions resulting from a mother's alcohol consumption during pregnancy, are a significant concern. The most severe form, fetal alcohol syndrome, is the most severe, causing abnormal appearances, poor coordination, low intelligence, behavior issues, hearing loss, and vision problems. Those affected are more likely to face school issues, legal issues, high-risk behaviors, and trouble with alcohol and recreational drug use. Fetal alcohol syndrome typically occurs when a pregnant woman drinks more than four drinks per day. The World Health Organization recommends avoiding alcohol entirely during pregnancy due to the unknown effects of even small amounts of alcohol. The World Health Organization emphasizes the need for a safe trimester for alcohol consumption.

3. **Raw or Unpasteurized Dairy**:

Explanation: Raw or unpasteurized dairy may carry harmful bacteria.

Illustration: Choose pasteurized milk, cheeses, and yogurts to reduce the risk.

Example: Greek yogurt with berries is a safe and nutritious dairy option.

4. **High Mercury Fish**:

Fish consumption during pregnancy is encouraged by European, Australian, and American guidelines due to its fat-containing properties, such as salmon and tuna, which contain essential fatty acids for fetal neurodevelopment. However, concerns about heavy metals' effects on fetal neurodevelopment have led many mothers to avoid eating fish. Current research suggests 2-3 servings of low-methyl mercury-containing fish per week during pregnancy are safe and beneficial. Mercury accumulates in fish through their diet, with higher-ups on the food chain having higher levels. Fish oil dietary supplements containing both EPA and DHA, or algae-derived DHA-only oils, are an alternative. A laboratory evaluation of 30 popular fish oil supplements found very low levels of mercury, far below the upper safety limit set by the Global Organization for EPA and DHA Omega-3s.

Explanation: Certain fish high in mercury can affect the baby's developing nervous system.

Illustration: Limit shark, swordfish, and king mackerel; choose low-mercury options.

Example: Grilled tilapia or salmon are excellent low-mercury fish choices.

5. **Processed and High-Sugar Foods**:

Explanation: Excessive processed and high-sugar foods can lead to unnecessary weight gain.

Illustration: Opt for whole foods and snacks like fruits, nuts, and vegetables.

Example: Sliced apples with peanut butter make a nutritious and satisfying snack.

The first trimester of pregnancy is a crucial period for a woman's health and well-being. It involves a delicate balance of nutrient intake and avoiding potential risks. Pregnancy brings emotional and physical changes, and taking care of oneself during this time can help the pregnancy go smoothly. The body is capable of providing the baby with what it needs, even when it struggles with eating or keeping food down. Prioritizing essential nutrients and making informed food choices can help expectant mothers lay a strong foundation for a healthy pregnancy. Eating healthy, moving the body, controlling stress, and getting enough rest are essential for a healthier pregnancy. Women carrying one baby may gain between 1 and 5 pounds during the first trimester, as long as they don't overeat. Consult a healthcare professional for personalized advice.

Chapter 2

**SAFEGUARDING THE SECOND
TRIMESTER**

Ensuring a healthy second trimester is vital for the well-being of both the expecting woman and the growing baby. In this critical period of pregnancy, let's explore the nutritional factors that contribute to the baby's healthy growth and development.

<u>Dietary Considerations for Growth and Development:</u>
1. **Diet High in Protein**:
Explanation: Babies' organs, muscles, and tissues grow in part because of proteins, the fundamental units of all life.
Case in point: Consume a diet rich in lean proteins such as chicken, fish, eggs, dairy, beans, and nuts.
A few examples of foods that are rich in protein are grilled chicken, lentils, and yogurt.

2. Intake of Folate:

Details: Folate aids in the prevention of birth abnormalities and is crucial for neural tube development.

Case in point: Consume leafy greens, citrus fruits, and fortified cereals for an appropriate folate consumption.

Examples: Folate and vitamin C are both found in spinach salads that include orange slices in them.

3. Calcium for Bone Development:

Explanation: Calcium aids in the development of the baby's bones and teeth.

Case in point: Incorporate dairy products, fortified plant-based milk, and leafy greens into your diet.

Example: A smoothie with yogurt, spinach, and almond milk is a calcium-rich option.

4. Iron-rich foods:

Explanation: Iron is vital for avoiding anemia and maintaining sufficient oxygen flow to the growing fetus.

Case in point: Choose red meat, poultry, fish, and iron-fortified grains.

Example: A stir-fry with lean meat, broccoli, and quinoa is a delightful iron-rich food.

5. Vitamin-Rich Adventures: A, C, and D:

Vitamins A, C, and D join the stage as crucial performers in the second-trimester drama. This part unveils a brilliant tapestry of vitamin-rich activities, examining colorful fruits and vegetables, sunshine exposure, and nutritional sources that contribute to maternal health and fetal growth. Readers go on a voyage of sensory pleasures that highlight the richness of vitamins.

<u>Reducing Risks Through Smart Food Choices:</u>

1. Limiting Mercury Exposure:

Explanation: High mercury levels may impair the baby's growing neurological system.

Case in point: Choose low-mercury seafood like salmon, shrimp, and trout over high-mercury types.

Example: Baked fish with lemon and herbs is a safe and healthy alternative.

2. Avoiding Raw or Undercooked Foods:

Explanation: Raw or undercooked meals may pose a risk of foodborne infections.

Case in point: Ensure all meats, eggs, and seafood are completely cooked.

Example: Opt for well-boiled eggs and completely cooked meats in meals.

3. Balancing Nutrient Intake:

Explanation: Maintaining a balanced diet is vital for general health and growth.

Case in point: Include a variety of fruits, vegetables, healthy grains, and proteins in each meal.

Example: Quinoa salad with mixed veggies and grilled chicken delivers a well-rounded lunch.

4. Hydration and herbal infusions:

Hydration has a leading role in lowering risks and enhancing overall health. This part covers the advantages of being well-hydrated throughout the second trimester and introduces herbal infusions that give both taste and sustenance. From refreshing mint to relaxing chamomile, readers are advised to establish hydration routines that contribute to a healthy and vibrant pregnancy experience.

In conclusion, protecting the second trimester entails a meticulous evaluation of food choices. By concentrating on a nutrient-rich diet and making sensible food choices, expecting moms may greatly contribute to the healthy growth and development of their newborns. Always speak with a healthcare expert for specialized advice tailored to your requirements.

Chapter 3

PRIORITIZING NUTRITION IN THE THIRD TRIMESTER

The third trimester represents the last stretch of pregnancy, and providing appropriate nutrition during this vital stage is essential for both the mother's well-being and the proper growth of the baby. Let's discuss the vital nutrients to prioritize and possible risks to avoid throughout late pregnancy.

<u>Essential Nutrients for Late Pregnancy</u>:
1. Calcium for Fetal Bone Growth:
Calcium is crucial for reinforcing skeletal growth during late pregnancy, and incorporating calcium-rich meals, such as dairy and fortified substitutes, into your diet can ensure a strong foundation for both maternal and fetal well-being. Vitamin D is also essential for bone health, and incorporating it into your diet can promote calcium absorption. Dairy products, fortified plant-based milk, and leafy greens are

recommended, as they provide calcium and necessary nutrients. Enjoy the healthy glow of vitamin D-rich foods.

2. Omega-3 Fatty Acids for Brain Development: Omega-3 fatty acids take center stage, supporting the growing brain and vision of the unborn child. From fatty fish to plant-based sources like flaxseeds, readers discover a variety of alternatives that deliver this critical mineral. The story builds a tale of sustenance, highlighting the necessity of omega-3s in the delicate tapestry of late pregnancy.

Explanation: Omega-3s, particularly DHA, are vital for the development of the baby's brain and eyes.

Illustration: Include fatty fish (like salmon), chia seeds, and walnuts in your diet.

Example: Baked salmon with quinoa and a side of steamed broccoli is a healthy omega-3-rich dinner.

3. Iron for Blood Support: In the nutritional symphony, iron gets a stage to support the

increased blood supply expected by late pregnancy. This section goes into the necessity of iron-rich diets, from lean meats to fortified cereals, ensuring that the mother's body is well-prepared for the demands of delivery. Expectant women embark on a journey that not only nourishes but also preserves energy in the latter months of pregnancy.

Explanation: Iron remains vital for avoiding anemia and sustaining the increased blood volume.

Illustration: Choose lean meats, beans, and iron-fortified cereals.

Example: A lentil and vegetable stew with lean meat delivers a robust iron boost.

4. Protein for Tissue Growth:

Explanation: Adequate protein intake aids the baby's tissue growth and development.

Case in point: Include sources including eggs, chicken, fish, and plant-based proteins.

Example: Grilled chicken with quinoa and roasted veggies is a protein-packed supper.

<u>**Identifying and Avoiding Potential Hazards:**</u>

1. Monitoring blood pressure:

Explanation: High blood pressure might offer hazards during the third trimester.

Case in point: Consume potassium-rich foods like bananas and oranges to help manage blood pressure.

Example: A fruit salad with banana slices and orange segments is a delightful and healthful alternative.

2. Limiting Sodium Intake:

Explanation: Excessive sodium may lead to fluid retention and elevated blood pressure.

Case in point: Choose fresh, healthy meals and minimize processed and high-sodium snacks.

Example: A handmade vegetable stir-fry with minimal additional salt is a low-sodium choice.

3. Monitoring Gestational Diabetes Risk:

Explanation: Late pregnancy raises the risk of gestational diabetes.

Case in point: Opt for complex carbs like whole grains and check sugar consumption.

Example: Quinoa salad with roasted sweet potatoes and chickpeas delivers a healthy, low-glycemic dinner.

4. Hydration and Edema Management:
Explanation: Adequate hydration helps control edema, particularly in the latter stages of pregnancy.
Case in point: Drink lots of water and eat hydrating foods like watermelon and cucumber.
Example: A pleasant watermelon and cucumber salad is a hydrating and healthy snack.

In conclusion, addressing nutrition in the third trimester entails a continuing emphasis on necessary nutrients and a watchful approach to possible dangers. By adopting educated food choices and paying attention to general well-being, pregnant moms may contribute to a healthy pregnancy. Always contact a healthcare professional for individualized advice based on specific requirements and circumstances.

Chapter 4

COMMON CULPRITS TO ELIMINATE

In this part, the attention is on the possible dangers connected with raw and unpasteurized items during pregnancy. From gourmet cheeses to specific deli meats, the chapter navigates the culinary scene, uncovering the threats presented by hazardous germs such as Listeria. Expectant moms are encouraged to exclude these probable causes from their diet to protect against foodborne infections that may pose dangers to both maternal and fetal health.

Eliminating some frequent offenders during pregnancy is vital to preserving both the mother and the growing baby. Let's review in depth the need to avoid raw and unpasteurized foodstuffs, high-mercury seafood, and the possible concerns linked to Listeria.

1. Raw and unpasteurized products:

Explanation: Consuming raw or unpasteurized items provides a considerable risk of bacterial contamination, perhaps leading to foodborne diseases that may be dangerous during pregnancy.

Case in point: Opt for pasteurized milk, cheeses, and juices to avoid the danger of hazardous germs like Salmonella and E. coli.

Examples: Choose pasteurized cheeses for sandwiches or snacks. Opt for pasteurized milk when cooking smoothies or porridge. Avoid ingesting raw or undercooked eggs in dishes like Caesar salad dressing.

2. Rich-Mercury Seafood and Fish: The story digs deep into the ocean of wise seafood selections, giving a guide to species that are low in mercury and rich in nutritional content. From salmon, a nutritional powerhouse, to shrimp and cod, readers find an assortment of alternatives that enable parents to experience the joys of the sea without sacrificing the well-being of themselves or their developing baby.

Explanation: High amounts of mercury in some seafood may significantly damage the baby's developing neurological system, making it vital to restrict or avoid specific fish during pregnancy.

Illustration: Focus on low-mercury choices to experience the advantages of omega-3 fatty acids without the accompanying hazards.

Examples: Choose low-mercury fish such as salmon, shrimp, and trout. Limit the intake of high-mercury seafood, including shark, swordfish, and king mackerel. Opt for canned light tuna instead of albacore tuna for a reduced mercury concentration.

3. Potential Listeria Hazards: The chapter unravels the tale of potential Listeria hazards, giving light on this silent culprit that presents special concerns during pregnancy. From deli foods to certain refrigerated smoked fish, expecting moms are escorted through a cautionary tale, highlighting the significance of removing these possible sources of Listeria from their diet.

Explanation: Listeria, a bacteria present in several foods, may lead to serious difficulties during pregnancy, including miscarriage or premature delivery.

Illustration: Practice food safety steps to limit the risk of Listeria infection and prioritize the intake of prepared and properly handled meals.

Examples: Avoid soft cheeses like feta, brie, and blue cheese unless they are labeled as pasteurized. Heat deli meats until they are boiling hot before ingesting. Be careful with refrigerated smoked fish and ensure it is thoroughly cooked before eating.

In conclusion, avoiding frequent offenders during pregnancy requires making smart dietary choices to limit the risk of foodborne diseases, mercury exposure, and Listeria contamination. By emphasizing food safety and selecting options that provide fewer hazards, pregnant moms may contribute to a healthier and safer pregnancy. Always speak with a healthcare expert for individualized advice based on your health and circumstances.

Chapter 5:

NAVIGATING DIETARY RESTRICTIONS

Navigating dietary limitations during pregnancy is a difficult path that requires a good grasp of foodborne diseases and the skill of identifying safe alternatives and substitutes. Let's investigate this sophisticated procedure in depth.

<u>Understanding Foodborne Illnesses:</u>
1. Listeria monocytogenes:
Explanation: Listeria is a bacteria that may lead to serious difficulties during pregnancy, including miscarriage or premature delivery.
Illustration: Be careful with high-risk meals, including soft cheeses, deli meats, and refrigerated smoked fish.
Example: Choose hard cheeses, heat deli meats, and fully prepare seafood to lessen the risk of Listeria.

2. Salmonella and E. coli:

Explanation: These bacteria may cause gastrointestinal difficulties and represent a danger to both the mother and the growing baby.

Case in point: Avoid raw or undercooked eggs, unpasteurized goods, and undercooked meats.

Example: Opt for pasteurized forms of milk and juices, ensuring meats and eggs are completely cooked.

3. Mercury in Seafood:

Explanation: High amounts of mercury in some fish may impair the baby's growing neurological system.

Illustration: Limit eating high-mercury seafood like shark and swordfish.

Example: Choose low-mercury alternatives like salmon and shrimp for vital omega-3 fatty acids.

<u>Safe Alternatives and Substitutions</u>:

1. Dairy Alternatives:

Explanation: For people with lactose sensitivity or following a vegan diet, there are various dairy replacements available.

Case in point: Opt for almond milk, soy milk, or oat milk as alternatives for regular dairy products.

Example: Use almond milk in smoothies or over cereal as a healthy alternative.

2. Protein Sources:

Explanation: Diversify protein sources to fit dietary constraints or preferences.

Case in point: Choose plant-based proteins such as beans, tofu, and tempeh.

Example: Lentil soup or a tofu stir-fry may supply protein without sacrificing nutritional goals.

3. Gluten-Free Grains:

Explanation: Those with gluten intolerance or celiac disease may try a range of gluten-free cereals.

Case in point: Embrace quinoa, rice, and gluten-free oats as alternatives to wheat-based items.

Example: Quinoa salad or gluten-free oatmeal may be tasty and safe alternatives.

4. Low-Sugar Substitutes:

Explanation: Managing sugar consumption is crucial for several health reasons, including gestational diabetes.

Case in point: Choose natural sweeteners like honey or maple syrup in moderation.

Example: Greek yogurt with a sprinkle of honey or a fruit compote delivers a delicious but balanced delight.

5. Managing Sodium Intake:

Explanation: High sodium levels may lead to fluid retention and high blood pressure, especially during pregnancy.

Illustration: Opt for fresh, natural meals and minimize the use of processed and high-sodium condiments.

Example: A handmade vegetable stir-fry with minimal additional salt gives a tasty, low-sodium option.

6. Catering to Vegetarian or Vegan Diets:

Explanation: Maintaining a vegetarian or vegan

diet during pregnancy demands careful monitoring of nutritional intake.

Case in point: Ensure adequate protein, iron, calcium, and vitamin B12 via plant-based foods and supplements.

Example: A lentil and vegetable curry with spinach and enriched nutritional yeast may provide critical nutrients.

7. Gluten-Free Options:

Explanation: Celiac illness or gluten sensitivity may entail avoiding gluten-containing cereals.

Case in point: Explore gluten-free options, including almond flour, coconut flour, and gluten-free pasta.

Example: Enjoy a gluten-free pasta salad with veggies and grilled chicken for a tasty and safe supper.

8. Balancing Carbohydrates for Gestational Diabetes:

Explanation: Managing carbohydrate consumption is critical for people coping with gestational diabetes.

Case in point: Choose complex carbs like whole grains, fruits, and vegetables for slow blood sugar release.

Example: Quinoa salad with roasted sweet potatoes and chickpeas delivers a healthy, low-glycemic dinner.

9. Hydration and Safe Beverages:

Explanation: Staying hydrated is crucial, but some beverages demand careful thought.

Illustration: Choose water as the main beverage and reduce caffeinated and sugary beverages.

Example: Infuse water with pieces of citrus fruits or berries for a delicious and naturally flavored alternative.

In negotiating dietary limitations during pregnancy, knowledge and ingenuity play crucial roles. Understanding the complexity of foodborne infections allows expecting mothers to make educated decisions. Embracing healthy alternatives and replacements promotes a broad and enjoyable diet, responding to individual requirements and interests. Always be in contact with healthcare specialists and nutritionists for individualized counseling suited to particular dietary limitations and health problems.

Chapter 6

MANAGING CRAVINGS AND AVERSIONS

Managing cravings and aversions during pregnancy is a delicate dance that takes a combination of inventiveness and nutritional expertise. Let's examine the art of managing pregnant urges and resolving aversions without sacrificing critical nourishment.

Balancing pregnancy cravings

Within the area of desires, the chapter gives insights into making good choices that fit with nutritional demands. Whether it's the need for a sweet pleasure or a savory snack, readers find alternatives and replacements that not only fulfill appetites but also contribute to the general health and well-being of both mother and baby. The story becomes a friend in navigating the lovely realm of pregnant cravings with awareness.

1. Understanding Cravings:

Explanation: Pregnancy cravings may vary from sweet to savory and may be impacted by hormonal changes.

Illustration: Embrace desires in moderation, concentrating on fulfilling them with healthier choices.

Example: Craving sweets? Opt for a modest dish of yogurt with fresh fruit or a piece of dark chocolate for a pleasant and healthy treat.

2. Diversifying Cravings:

Explanation: Encourage a range of desires to guarantee a well-rounded nutritional intake.

Illustration: If you desire something salty, balance it with a side of fresh veggies or a handful of almonds for increased nourishment.

Example: Pairing a modest portion of pretzels with hummus offers a balanced and enjoyable snack.

Addressing Aversions Without Compromising Nutrition:

1. Understanding Aversions: The story switches to addressing the issues of aversions, presenting a sympathetic investigation of the foods that may be encountered with resistance during pregnancy. From identifying the underlying causes of aversions to navigating suitable alternatives, pregnant moms are taken through a sophisticated path of resolving aversions without sacrificing nutritional demands.

Explanation: Aversions to specific meals may emerge owing to heightened senses or changes in taste perception during pregnancy.

Illustration: Find alternate nutrition sources that correspond with current tastes to maintain a balanced diet.

Example: If you are adverse to the flavor of meat, seek plant-based protein alternatives like tofu, beans, or lentils.

2. Creative Cooking Techniques:

Explanation: Experiment with different cooking techniques to make disagreeable meals more appealing.

Illustration: Roasting or grilling veggies may increase taste and texture, making them more attractive.

Example: If opposed to raw veggies, try roasted Brussels sprouts with a dab of balsamic sauce for a delightful variation.

3. Incorporating Strong Flavors:

Explanation: Introduce strong, tasty substances to conceal the taste of disagreeable meals.

Illustration: Use herbs, spices, and citrus to improve the flavor of foods and make them more pleasurable.

Example: A citrus-infused marinade may modify the flavor of fish, making it more palatable to individuals with aversions.

Personalized Nutritional Strategies:

1. Communication with Healthcare Professionals:

Explanation: Openly discuss urges and aversions with healthcare specialists for individualized assistance.

Illustration: Healthcare practitioners might offer supplements or alternative nutritional sources to address particular difficulties.

Example: If opposed to dairy, a healthcare expert may prescribe calcium-fortified plant-based milk.

2. Embracing the Power of Variety:

Explanation: A diversified diet helps guarantee that, even with aversions, nutritional demands are addressed.

Illustration: Explore a broad selection of cuisines to identify alternatives that suit existing tastes.

Example: If you are adverse to one kind of fruit, try a range of others to maintain a well-rounded fruit consumption.

Listening to the body's signals:

1. Intuitive Eating:
Explanation: Embrace intuitive eating by understanding and reacting to the body's cues for hunger and fullness.
Illustration: Avoid tight eating rules and instead tune in to what the body actually desires and needs.
Example: If feeling hungry between meals, go for a balanced snack like Greek yogurt with berries to satisfy cravings while nourishing the body.

Connecting with Other Expectant Mothers:

1. Community Support:
Explanation: Joining pregnant support groups or online communities enables the sharing of experiences and solutions for controlling cravings and aversions.

Illustration: Learn from people who have handled similar issues and learn innovative strategies to integrate a range of meals.

Example: Engaging in conversations about favorite pregnancy-friendly dishes or snacks may bring inspiration and practical recommendations.

In conclusion, controlling cravings and aversions throughout pregnancy is a continuous process that needs both flexibility and ingenuity. By recognizing the underlying causes of cravings and aversions and adopting a range of nutrient-rich options, pregnant women may find a balance that delights their taste buds while guaranteeing appropriate nutrition. Always speak with healthcare specialists for specific counsel tailored to particular requirements and circumstances.

Chapter 7

DINING OUT AND SOCIAL SITUATIONS

Navigating eating out and social settings during pregnancy demands a combination of educated decision-making and efficient communication to ensure both gastronomic satisfaction and nutritional requirements are addressed. Let's discuss ways to make educated decisions outside the home and express dietary demands successfully.

<u>Making informed choices beyond home</u>:
1. Researching menus in advance:
Explanation: Prior to going out, examine restaurant menus online to locate pregnancy-friendly selections.
Illustration: Look for foods rich in critical nutrients and low in possible dangers, such as undercooked or uncooked ingredients.
Example: Opt for grilled chicken salads, well-cooked pasta meals, or vegetarian alternatives with a range of vibrant veggies.

2. Choosing Pregnancy-Friendly Cuisines:

Explanation: Explore cuisines recognized for their focus on well-cooked, tasty ingredients, such as Mediterranean or Japanese cuisine.

Illustration: These cuisines frequently provide a range of nutrient-rich alternatives with lesser risks of foodborne diseases.

Example: Sushi rolls with cooked fish or vegetable stir-fries may be delightful and safe alternatives.

Communicating Dietary needs effectively:

The story changes to the significance of discussing dietary demands successfully in social circumstances. Whether at a family gathering or a meal with friends, pregnant moms are encouraged to communicate their demands with confidence, creating an environment where their dietary requirements are acknowledged. The chapter provides a guide to assertiveness, ensuring that dietary decisions are expressed successfully without sacrificing the pleasure of social situations.

1. Clear and concise communication:

Explanation: Clearly convey dietary demands and limits to servers, stressing the significance of avoiding particular substances or cooking techniques.

Illustration: Use plain language and emphasize the desire for well-cooked dishes.

Example: Politely request, "Could you please ensure that my chicken is well-cooked, and I'd like to avoid any raw or undercooked ingredients?"

2. Customizing Menu Options:

Explanation: Don't hesitate to ask for tweaks or substitutes to accord with dietary preferences or aversions.

Illustration: Many restaurants are prepared to accept requests for ingredient substitutions or adjustments to cooking processes.

Example: Requesting a grilled chicken choice instead of fried or asking for a different side dish might modify the meal to meet dietary restrictions.

Selecting Safe Beverage Options

1. Avoiding Risky Beverages:

Explanation: Be careful with beverage selections, avoiding unpasteurized beverages or those with high caffeine levels.

Illustration: Opt for water, herbal teas, or pasteurized fruit juices as healthy and refreshing alternatives.

Example: sparkling water with a dash of fruit juice or a caffeine-free herbal tea may enhance the meal without sacrificing health.

Being Prepared for Unforeseen Circumstances:

1. Emergency Snack Kit:

Explanation: Carry a small kit with pregnancy-friendly snacks to ensure you have a nutritional choice if eating options are restricted.

Illustration: Pack foods like almonds, dried fruits, or granola bars to alleviate hunger in case of unforeseen delays or restricted meal alternatives.

Example: A handful of nuts or a piece of fruit from your pack may be a lifesaver in circumstances where adequate food may be rare.

Seeking support from dining companions:
1. Educating Friends and Family:
Explanation: Inform your dining partners about your dietary preferences and limits to develop understanding and support.
Illustration: Share information about your cuisine preferences and any unique issues to facilitate a joint effort in picking acceptable eating alternatives.
Example: Communicate with friends: "I'm avoiding certain meals for the baby's health. I'd appreciate your aid in selecting a location with variety and well-cooked selections."

Embracing the Culinary Experience:
1. Focusing on Enjoyment:
Explanation: While being attentive to dietary restrictions, cherish the meal experience and concentrate on enjoying the company of friends or family.

Illustration: Balance nutritional concerns with the joy of eating new meals or indulging in occasional pleasures.

Example: Share a dessert with the table or enjoy a modest treat as a part of the entire culinary experience.

In summary, handling eating out and social settings during pregnancy takes a mix of thoughtful decision-making and excellent communication. By studying menus, expressing needs clearly, and being prepared for unanticipated events, expecting moms may enjoy a variety of eating experiences while prioritizing their health and nutritional requirements. Always speak with healthcare experts for individualized advice based on specific requirements and circumstances.

Chapter 8

FREQUENTLY ASKED QUESTIONS

Expert Insights on Common Concerns

Chapter 8 provides a guide to unwinding the strands of misinformation that commonly weave through the fabric of pregnancy. Expert voices deconstruct misunderstandings around particular meals, workout regimens, and common beliefs, helping readers to make educated choices based on factual and evidence-based information. The tale becomes a beacon of clarity, debunking beliefs that may add to unwarranted fears throughout this transforming journey.

1. Can I exercise during pregnancy?
Expert Insight: Exercise is typically suggested during pregnancy, but it's crucial to talk with your healthcare professional. Low-impact exercises like walking, swimming, or prenatal yoga are typically excellent for maintaining fitness and overall well-being.

2. What Should I Eat to Ensure a Healthy Pregnancy?

Expert Insight: A well-balanced diet is vital. Focus on a mix of fruits, vegetables, lean meats, nutritious grains, and dairy or dairy substitutes. Consult with a nutritionist for specialized guidance on addressing particular nutritional demands during pregnancy.

3. How Much Weight Should I Gain During Pregnancy?

Expert Insight: Weight gain guidelines differ depending on pre-pregnancy BMI. Generally, it varies from 25 to 35 pounds for a healthy BMI. However, specific situations may require alternative goals. Consult with your healthcare physician for tailored guidance.

4. Is It Safe to Travel During Pregnancy?

Expert Insight: In most circumstances, it's safe to travel during pregnancy, particularly in the early and mid-stages. However, contact your healthcare practitioner, especially if you develop issues or are nearing your due date. Stay hydrated and take breaks to stretch during lengthy flights.

Common Concerns About Foods to Avoid

1. Raw Seafood:

Question: Can I consume sushi or other raw seafood during pregnancy?

Expert Insight: It's suggested to avoid raw seafood during pregnancy owing to the danger of foodborne infections like Salmonella or Listeria. Opt for prepared fish selections to guarantee safety.

2. Soft Cheeses:

Question: Are soft cheeses safe to consume when pregnant?

Expert Insight: Some soft cheeses may host hazardous germs like Listeria. It's best to buy pasteurized versions and avoid variations like Brie and Camembert.

3. Deli Meats:

Question: Can I consume deli meats during pregnancy?

Expert Insight: Deli meats may involve the risk of Listeria infection. It's safer to heat them until steaming to eradicate possible microorganisms before ingestion.

4. High-Mercury Fish:
Question: Which fish should I avoid owing to their high mercury content?
Expert Insight: Fish such as shark, swordfish, king mackerel, and tilefish have high mercury levels, which might be dangerous during pregnancy. Opt for low-mercury options like salmon and shrimp.

5. Caffeine Intake:
Question: How much caffeine is safe during pregnancy?
Expert Insight: High caffeine consumption has been related to an increased risk of miscarriage. It's typically suggested to restrict caffeine to 200 mg per day, comparable to around one 12-ounce cup of coffee.

Misconceptions about Pregnancy Nutrition

1. "Eating for Two":

Misconception: Should I eat double quantities if I'm "eating for two"?

Expert Insight: While nutritional demands rise, doubling quantities may contribute to excessive weight gain. Focus on nutrient-dense foods rather than quantity.

2. Artificial Sweeteners:

Misconception: Are artificial sweeteners safe during pregnancy?

Expert Insight: Most artificial sweeteners are deemed safe in moderation. However, it's necessary to talk with a healthcare expert regarding unique situations.

3. Spicy Meals and Heartburn:

Misconception: Should I Avoid Spicy Meals to Prevent Heartburn During Pregnancy?

Expert Insight: Spicy meals don't uniformly induce heartburn. Experimenting with various meals and meal schedules might help alleviate pain.

4. Vegetarian or Vegan Diets:

Misconception: Is it healthy to adopt a vegetarian or vegan diet during pregnancy?

Expert Insight: With appropriate preparation, vegetarian and vegan diets may supply enough nutrients throughout pregnancy. Consult a healthcare practitioner for individualized counseling.

5. Cravings Indicating Nutrient Deficiencies:

Misconception: Do certain appetites indicate dietary deficiencies?

Expert Insight: Cravings are normal throughout pregnancy and don't always signal shortages. It's vital to maintain a balanced diet for general well-being.

<u>Addressing Myths and Misconceptions</u>:

1. Myth: Eating for Two Means Eating Twice as Much.

Expert Insight: This is a widespread misperception. While nutritional demands rise during pregnancy, the focus should be on nutrient-dense meals rather than doubling the amount. Quality over quantity is crucial.

2. Myth: Avoid all seafood during pregnancy.
Expert Insight: Not true. While high-mercury seafood should be avoided, low-mercury choices like salmon and shrimp are rich in omega-3 fatty acids, which are crucial for embryonic brain development. Enjoy seafood in moderation and pick carefully.

3. Myth: Exercise Can Harm the Baby.
Expert Insight: Exercise is typically safe and useful throughout pregnancy. It may aid with mood, energy levels, and general wellness. However, some high-risk situations may demand changes, so always talk with your healthcare professional before beginning or maintaining an exercise plan.

4. Myth: Morning sickness only happens in the morning.
Expert Insight: Morning sickness may come at any moment of the day. Its severity varies across

people. Eating small, regular meals, keeping hydrated, and getting adequate rest may help reduce nausea.

5. Myth: All herbal teas are safe during pregnancy.
Expert Insight: Not all herbal teas are safe. Some herbs may have detrimental effects on pregnancy. Avoid teas with components like licorice root, chamomile, or excessive caffeine. Consult with your healthcare physician for a list of safe herbal teas.

6. Myth: A high heart rate during exercise is dangerous.
Expert Insight: While it's vital to monitor heart rate during exercise, a slight rise is typically harmless. Focus on perceived effort and the capacity to carry on a conversation. If in doubt, speak with your healthcare practitioner for tailored counsel.

Providing additional guidance:

1. Staying Hydrated:

Expert Insight: Adequate hydration is vital throughout pregnancy. It helps maintain amniotic fluid, improves nutrition delivery, and reduces dehydration-related problems. Aim for at least 8–10 glasses of water every day.

2. Monitoring Kick Counts:

Expert Insight: In the latter stages of pregnancy, tracking fetal movements, known as kick counts, may give comfort about the baby's well-being. If you see a severe reduction in movement, contact your healthcare professional.

3. Handling Stress:

Expert Insight: Managing stress is vital for both mother and fetal well-being. Techniques like deep breathing, prenatal yoga, and mindfulness may help decrease stress. Consult with your healthcare practitioner if stress gets unbearable.

4. Choosing a Birth Plan:

Expert Insight: Discussing birth planning with your healthcare practitioner is vital. Consider issues including pain treatment alternatives, birth preferences, and probable problems. Flexibility is crucial since birth plans may require revisions depending on circumstances.

5. Preparing for Breastfeeding:

Expert Insight: Attend breastfeeding courses, get guidance from lactation consultants, and establish a friendly atmosphere for nursing. Understanding good latch methods and having a breastfeeding-friendly location may increase the nursing experience.

Remember, individual experiences may vary, and it's vital to speak with healthcare specialists for specialized recommendations suited to your unique circumstances. Always reach out to your healthcare practitioner with any concerns or questions throughout pregnancy.

Coping with Sleep Disturbances:

1. Is it normal to have trouble sleeping during pregnancy?

Expert Insight: Yes, sleep difficulties are frequent. As the pregnancy continues, pain, frequent urination, and hormonal changes might disrupt sleep. Establish a calm nighttime routine, utilize pillows for support, and discuss sleep difficulties with your healthcare professional.

2. Can I Sleep on My Back?

Expert Insight: While resting on your back is typically safe in the early stages of pregnancy, it's encouraged to sleep on your side later on to optimize blood flow to the uterus. Use cushions for support, and consider a pregnant pillow for enhanced comfort.

Managing Swelling and Discomfort:

1. Why Am I Swelling, and When Should I Be Concerned?

Expert Insight: Swelling, or edema, is prevalent owing to increased blood volume and fluid retention. However, rapid or significant swelling might suggest a concern. Contact your healthcare practitioner if you detect considerable swelling in the hands, face, or feet, particularly if accompanied by other symptoms.

2. How Can I Alleviate Back Pain During Pregnancy?Expert Insight: Back discomfort is prevalent owing to the changing of the body's center of gravity. Practice proper posture, utilize supportive seats, and participate in activities prescribed by your healthcare physician. Prenatal yoga or swimming may also help ease back pain.

Preparing for Labor and Delivery:
1. When Should I Go to the Hospital During Labor?
Expert Insight: Contact your healthcare practitioner to decide when to go to the hospital. Generally, proceed to the hospital when contractions are regular, powerful, and approximately five minutes apart. If your water breaks or if you encounter any problems, seek medical attention soon.

2. What pain relief options are available during labor?

Expert Insight: Pain alleviation treatments differ. Discuss your preferences with your healthcare professional and examine choices like epidurals, breathing techniques, hydrotherapy, or other pain treatment approaches. Be flexible and prepared to modify depending on the course of labor.

Postpartum Concerns:

1. How Can I Support Mental Health Postpartum?

Expert Insight: Postpartum mental wellness is vital. Seek support from loved ones, explore therapy if required, and talk freely about your emotions. If you have signs of postpartum depression or anxiety, contact your healthcare practitioner for help and assistance.

2. What Can I Expect Regarding Postpartum Recovery?

Expert Insight: Postpartum recovery varies, but frequent occurrences include uterine contractions, vaginal bleeding (lochia), and changes in mood. Rest, a good diet, and light workouts as allowed by your healthcare professional may assist in a smoother recovery.

Remember that every pregnancy is unique, and individual experiences may differ. Always speak with your healthcare practitioner for individualized advice based on your unique health condition and circumstances. Regular prenatal check-ups allow you the opportunity to address concerns and get advice throughout your pregnancy.

CONCLUSION
EMPOWERING A HEALTHY PREGNANCY

Recapitulating Key Guidelines for an Empowered Pregnancy:

1. Regular prenatal check-ups:
Guideline: Schedule and attend frequent prenatal check-ups to assess both your health and the baby's progress. These check-ups enable healthcare experts to address issues, give direction, and guarantee a safe pregnancy.

2. Balanced Nutrition:
Guidelines: Embrace a well-balanced diet rich in fruits, vegetables, lean meats, whole grains, and dairy or dairy substitutes. Prioritize vital nutrients, including folic acid, iron, calcium, and omega-3 fatty acids, for optimum fetal growth.

3. Adequate Hydration:
Guidelines: Stay hydrated by drinking lots of water throughout the day. Proper hydration

promotes amniotic fluid levels, assists digestion, and helps reduce typical pregnant discomforts like constipation.

4. Regular Exercise:
Guidelines: Engage in regular, moderate exercise unless instructed differently by your healthcare physician. Activities such as walking, swimming, and prenatal yoga help boost general well-being, control weight, and encourage a gentler delivery experience.

5. Adequate Rest and Sleep:
Guidelines: Prioritize appropriate rest and quality sleep. Create a pleasant sleep environment, develop a nighttime routine, and consider napping when required to enhance both physical and emotional well-being.

6. Stress Management:
Guidelines: Implement stress-reduction practices such as deep breathing, meditation, or prenatal massages. Managing stress is crucial for mother

health and leads to a pleasant pregnancy experience.

<u>Celebrating a Nutritionally Sound Pregnancy Journey</u>

1. Educational Empowerment:
Celebration: Celebrate your dedication to educating yourself about pregnancy nutrition. Understanding the significance of different nutrients helps you make educated dietary choices that favorably benefit both your health and the baby's growth.

2. Culinary Exploration:
Celebration: Embrace the delight of culinary discovery by exploring new recipes and introducing a varied variety of tastes and textures into your meals. Celebrate the chance to nurture yourself and your baby with a range of nutrient-dense meals.

3. Body Appreciation:

Celebration: Celebrate the changes in your body as it adjusts to support the developing life inside. Appreciate the power and tenacity of your body throughout the pregnancy journey, seeing it as a vehicle for the wondrous process of generating life.

4. Connection with the infant:
Celebration: Foster a strong connection with your infant through mindful activities. Take pauses to feel their movements, chat with them, and participate in activities that increase the emotional relationship between you and your developing child.

5. Community Support:
Celebration: Celebrate the support and encouragement received from your spouse, family, friends, and healthcare professionals. Surround yourself with a positive community that uplifts and adds to a caring atmosphere.

6. Preparation for Parenthood:

Celebration: Acknowledge the measures taken to prepare for parenting, including attending prenatal courses, reading informed literature, and actively engaging in conversations about birth planning and postpartum care. Each effort adds to an easier transition into parenting.

Creating lasting memories:
1. Documenting the Journey:
Memorable Act: Celebrate the adventure by photographing crucial events. Keep a pregnancy notebook, snap photographs, and document the feelings and milestones that make this time special. These memories will become treasured recollections for both you and your child.

2. Bonding Activities:
Memorable Act: Engage in bonding activities with your spouse and loved ones. Attend prenatal courses together, engage in baby showers, and build rituals that deepen the emotional bonds within your expanding family.

Preparing a Nurturing Environment:

1. Nesting Rituals:

Nurturing Act: Embrace nesting habits to establish a loving atmosphere at home. Set up the baby's nursery, arrange infant needs, and imbue the area with warmth and affection. This preparation helps create a feeling of preparedness for the forthcoming arrival.

2. Connection with Nature:

Nurturing Act: Spend time in nature, whether it's on leisurely hikes at a local park or just enjoying the fresh air in your garden. Connecting with nature fosters a feeling of relaxation and tranquility, benefiting both your mental and emotional well-being.

Celebrating the Journey Together:

1. Maternity Photoshoot:

Joyful Act: Consider maternity photography to capture the beauty and pleasure of this unique time. Celebrate your changing body and the anticipation of a new life. The images serve as a physical reminder of the love and joy surrounding your pregnancy.

2. Celebratory Gatherings:
Joyful Act: Host or attend celebratory gatherings with friends and family. Share the excitement of imminent fatherhood, get well wishes, and rejoice in the love and support that surrounds you. Celebrations build lasting memories of this crucial life step.

As you continue to enjoy the powerful adventure of pregnancy, remember that each act of celebration, care, and contemplation adds to a comprehensive and rewarding experience. Cherish the times, emphasize self-care, and look forward to the great journey that lies ahead as you bring a new life into the world.

9 7 9 8 8 7 4 4 1 2 5 2 4